I0766817

YOUR PERSONAL HYPERTROPHY WORKOUT PLAN

THE 12 ATHLETIC WEEKS OF HERCULES

FULL PRACTICE BULKING PLAN, NUTRITION TIPS, STRETCHES, EXTRA DELOAD WEEK

Copyright © 2019 by Achilleas Karakatsanis. All Rights Reserved

No part of this publication may be reproduced, distributed, or transmitted in any form or by any means, including photocopying, recording, or other electronic or mechanical methods, or by any information storage and retrieval system without the prior written permission of the publisher, except in the case of very brief quotations embodied in critical reviews and certain other noncommercial uses permitted by copyright law.

Disclaimer

Exercise is inherently strenuous and potentially dangerous. Consult your physician before starting any exercise program. Achilleas Karakatsanis is not responsible for injuries or health problems incurred as a result of exercise or related advice.

ISBN: 9781796528909

TABLE OF CONTENTS

CHAPTER ONE

MACRONUTRIENTS AND DIETARY SUPPLEMENTS

INTRODUCTION TO THE COMPONENTS OF A BALANCED NUTRITION AND TRAINING

DIETARY SUPPLEMENTS:

You take supplements if you cannot have food ready from home. If you manage to have a balanced diet, then you do not need more protein in a Shake. You will need creatine and omega-3 fat, zma (B12, zinc and magnesium) and a lot of water when you reach a satisfactory level. In the winter when I start my bulk trainings because I have free time and I can cook, I take no protein supplements. Only some of the ones I will mention below.

When my macronutrients are complete, I don't need to 'load' my body with more protein. Besides, when you want to put on weight you have to increase your carbohydrates and fats relative to protein. Protein is 1.4-1.8g per kilos of bodyweight, the carbohydrates is 4-4.2g, and the fats is 1.2-1.5g.

You do not need to study much more of them, but to be consistent and disciplined towards training, nutrition and above all, yourself.

Remember that your health comes before your image in the mirror and the weights you want to lift with your arms or chest or legs.

Let's put them in order in your mind.

PROTEIN:

4 CALORIES PER GRAM.

The most widespread supplement and perhaps the most mythical one. You get a protein Shake and you just become huge. Veins pumping from everywhere, your chest or butt pops out and you are ready to destroy the entire gym with your power. And suddenly you take protein before training and your workouts are the same! You take some every time before and after but you don't become huge. Maybe it's the brand's fault. I'll find another. But you forget something very important: protein is a macronutrient that helps build the muscle fibers 'injured' by training. It is also a good source of energy for your workouts if you manage to "burn" all the glycogen stores on your liver and muscles. Which in their entirety is 500 gr. With 4 calories per 1g, carbohydrates alone in our body account for 2000 calories. A lot, right? However, they are needed to provide us with all the movements we do every day. Not just to lift in the gym, but also climb the stairs, walk, lift groceries, open a door, move our hands or feet, etc., but let me continue on the protein...

A basic macronutrient ingredient that contributes to the good functioning of our muscles and also to our _better_ recovery. Watch out! _Better_, not faster! No supplement does wonders, because it's simply a "supplement". It's a food substitute. They are not performance enhancing drugs or androgens.

So, we need protein right after training so it can do its job of repairing the injured muscles. And in the remaining meals until we sleep, we need more carbohydrates and protein at the same level (40g-60g/meal).

CARBOHYDRATES:

4 CALORIES PER GRAM.

Carbohydrates are the most important source of energy in our bodies. When we deal with anything in our daily lives that changes the length of our muscles, we consume carbohydrates from the liver's stores (first store) and then the muscle glycogen (second store). That's why it's important to have a good amount of carbohydrates in our diet. Carbohydrates are among the most important macronutrients because they contribute to the smooth functioning of the muscles and most of our body's functions.

FATS:

9 CALORIES PER GRAM.

Fat, besides fat around the waist, also contributes as a thermostat to our body. With fat, water and blood the temperature of our body is regulated. With fat we also draw energy for our workouts when glycogen stores run out.

It is good to have a percentage around 10% to 16% in our body when we want to gain muscle weight but also when we want to lose weight. In essence, when we gain weight we will put on lean mass as well as fat.

It is inevitable. Just as when we lose weight, we lose both fat and muscular mass. Just with the right diet and exercise we will keep it at the rates it was before, until the end of our workouts.

HYDRATION:

1 TO 2 LITRES PER DAY.

Water is a very important factor in both sports and nutrition. The greatest percentage in our body as well as in our muscles is water. For this reason, we need to drink enough water to be hydrated throughout our day and during our workouts. For this reason, we also need to consume sodium (salt). Because salt does fluid retention in our body and uses it when our body needs it.

To give you a picture of your muscles I will explain what they have inside:

• Protein (18%)

• Fat (5%)

• Carbohydrates (1%)

• Vitamins and minerals (1%)

• Water (75%)

Therefore, we understand that water is very important for our training as well as for our body in general. It also helps as perform better our workouts. If we are dehydrated we will perform poor. Below we have a table that helps you learn how much water you need according to your weight:

So, per 5 kilos of bodyweight, we add 0.2 liter of water per day.

Kilos	Liters of Water
45	1.9
50	2.1
55	2.3
60	2.5
65	2.7
70	2.9
75	3.1
80	3.3
85	3.5

ALCOHOL AND JUNK FOOD:

7 and 9 CALORIES PER GRAM.

Alcohol and junk food contain the most calories. That's why it's reasonable to have junk food or a drink once a week. Apart from the fact that the macronutrients of junk food are deficient in terms of quality (protein, fiber) and too much in terms of fats, simple and complex carbohydrates. The protein they contain is minimal or equal sometimes but not of the same biological value. That way, our body absorbs much less macronutrients because it does not recognize the ingredients that fall into our stomach. That's why much caution is needed when we eat out. We may need to eat more some days (1-2 times a week) but it would be good to be careful what we EAT.

OMEGA 3 AND 6 FATS:

MICRONUTRIENTS.

Omega 3 and 6 fatty acids help your body and especially the muscles to recover better. Not faster, _better_! Omega fats are known to provide better muscle performance and recovery. They also help with brain function and better performance of our immune system. For this, it is important to eat fatty fish foods. If you don't have the time to cook fish, then an omega 3 or 6 supplement would be very good for your diet. Within 10 days you will see the difference on how your body responds after the training and the following days. Your feet or back may hurt the day after training but remember, that's a good sign. Three (3) capsules per day is the recommended dose and should not be exceeded. One capsule after your meal.

CREATINE*:

Creatine or phosphocreatine is the body's fuel during the first 10 seconds of exercise. It increases performance by 10-15% on single or repeated short (up to 30 seconds) maximum efforts. It is the fastest form of 'fuel' since it is consumed very quickly but it brings a lot of energy to our muscles. For this reason, a supplement of creatine is important. Which is the purest supplement on the market right now. Nothing bad happens if you take it and our body absorbs it right away. But we need to take it because we can't store too much. 5g per day before the training is enough to give you explosiveness between sets and to help you fill up your energy in less time than the one indicated in each training session. It is such a pure supplement that does not need either 'charging' or loading circles. You can start and stop it immediately. Professional bodybuilders stop it when they are in a weight losing period because the creatine hydrates our muscles. Because water in performance and in the recovery of muscles is very important. And surely these athletes do not want a hint of water on their bodies during the days of the contest. It has an anabolic effect (muscle growth) when combined with strength training. Also, possible injury prevention and improved immune function exist. So, let's learn from the example.

*No serious side effects from long-term use have been reported.

MULTIVITAMINS:

Multivitamins are suggested to people who can't manage to get their vitamins from food and do not get to eat fruits and vegetables. Once a day is enough to contribute to good concentration and increase our energy levels.

1 to 2 capsules depending on our nutritional needs.

ZMA:

Zma is a vitamin supplement with zinc, magnesium and vitamin B12. All three offer better recovery of injured muscle fibers while resting in our sleep. They greatly contribute to the proper functioning of our organs, our immune system and our bones. 2-3 capsules 2 hours before sleep on an empty stomach. Do not consume dairy products before zma, as they break down vitamin function.

BRANCH-CHAINED AMINO ACIDS (BCAAS):

Bcaas are the essential amino acids leucine, isoleucine, valine. The combination of these amino acids makes up about 1/3 of the skeletal muscle tissue. After training, the bcaas put the body in an increased hypertrophic state by increasing protein composition. Bcaas are metabolised within the muscle cell and not in the liver. This means they are more likely to be used for muscle synthesis than as a fuel for energy.

FRUIT AND VEGETABLES:

It is important to eat fruit and vegetables because they give us their vitamins and their plant fibers. Besides that, they help us with our cravings for sweets and keeps our stomach full for at least a while. Fruit consumption is suggested one hour before eating and not after, because the fructose contained in them makes digestion after a meal difficult. Vegetables should be consumed in our meals as follows:

- In the bulk phase we eat our meal and then the vegetables or somewhat along with the meal.

- In the weight loss phase, we eat vegetables first and then our meal.

- Vegetables, because of the fibers and the carbohydrates contained in them, make us feel fuller.

- In the phase we are now, we consume our vegetables after or alongside our lunch and fruits before our meal or after training.

REST:

Rest is one of our most important priorities in our workouts and muscle hypertrophy. It helps to recover muscles injured during training and to redistribute energy stores in our body until the next training. The more rested we are, the more efficient we will be and the more we will benefit from muscle hypertrophy. Maybe you don't understand how important it is now, but in the long run you will realise that without rest we cannot have beautiful results. Everything must be in harmony to have better results. You can't do a little of everything and get the best results. You can't eat a little and expect to be full. Just as you can't eat a lot and expect to lose weight. Just remember how important resting and sleeping 7 to 9 hours a day is:

- Faster recovery of our muscles.

- Increased levels of testosterone and growth hormone.

- More energy for your workouts.

- Sleep reduces cortisol levels in our body.

But let's talk about what you're thinking. What is this cortisol? Surely, it's not some bug spray.

In a few words, cortisol is the hormone of anxiety.
It causes many problems in our body with some of them being the following:

- loss of muscle mass
- weakening of our immune system
- hyperglycaemia
- In large proportions it leads to minimal wound healing

Cortisol is essential for our body to produce epinephrine. However, when produced in large proportions, it has very bad effects on our body. So, it's good to try to keep it under control as much as we can.

MEAL FREQUENCY:

Big issue, I know! The frequency of meals is something that depends on the person. During the day you have a calorie limit to consume. Let's say 2000 calories. The least would be in 4 meals. From then on, you can have as many meals as you want or whatever makes you feel full throughout your day. For example, I do 7 to 8 meals a day. Arnold Schwarzenegger did 5 meals a day when he wanted to gain weight. The amount of meals you do depends on your appetite and whether it keeps you full during the day. So, there is no right and wrong. Just remember to eat a regular meal 2-3 hours before training or fruit and protein 1-2 hours before and after training to take your protein and have a meal 1-2 hours after that. So set your diet right around your workouts, and then see how your body reacts to the meals of the day. At least 4 meals during the day if you want to get good results. And one after your training. Not immediately after it. Let one hour pass and then eat your meal.

FREQUENCY OF TRAINING:

The best for last! Workout frequency has to do with how many times you want to train your muscle groups. The best is to train each muscle group twice a week. That way, we contribute more to muscle hypertrophy and we have better results. In our program we have combined at least 5 trainings in the hypertrophy weeks and 3-4 trainings per week for strength weeks. Strength is important for hypertrophy because it makes us stronger so we can lift more in the weeks of hypertrophy, in a few wise words. The best training protocol is 6 days a week with the two training sessions being strength.

4 to 6 workouts per week.

Depending on our schedule, we can also do three cyclical trainings per week in a two-session protocol as follows:

1st week: upper - lower - upper

2nd week: lower - upper - lower

And it goes on alternately for as long as we want. Exercises can change every 4 to 6 weeks.

Our trainings can be in the morning or afternoon depending on each person's schedule. We do not suggest very early workouts because the spinal cord discs are hydrated and will be more unstable and charged with weight in the morning if you try to weight train. As time passes, the water stored during sleep is lost and the spine has more stability to better respond to strength training or even hypertrophy.

Do not forget to train your body 3 to 5 times a week. The week has 168 hours. You have to take 5 to 8 of them to exercise your body as best as you can and train like Hercules!

Stay tuned to our page at Instagram at the end of this book because we will upload more trainings for hypertrophy with protocols that help people who work and have few hours for training per week.

POWER, VISION & DISCIPLINE.

CHAPTER TWO

DAILY CALORIE INTAKE

INTRODUCTION TO THE COMPONENTS OF A BALANCED NUTRITION AND TRAINING

LET'S CHECK SOMETHING BASIC OUT:

Training is when you have a goal to lose or gain weight. Training is organised. Has a beginning and an End. When you know what exercises you will be doing and why, you are going to train. When you go to the gym without a goal, without knowing what you want to exercise, what the purpose of your workouts is and the only thing you do is exercise the mirror muscles (chest, arms, back) then you just workout. You don't train or do sports.

Below are some tips necessary for you to be a right and moral athlete in the gym. You must be right about your training but also as an Athlete or Trainee:

• Everyone believes that others are watching us when we work-out. Don't know about everyone but most of us think about it a lot! And everyone has the same attitude as we do. So, no one is looking at anyone. So, don't worry about what people think of you. Do your workout and do what you have to do.

• Do not mess around with your phone and leave the machines in each set.

• Always leave the space you used clean (benches, machines, mattresses, etc.)

• Re-Rack the Weights. ALWAYS!

• Do not bother anyone in the middle of a set.

• Do not waste time in the locker room .

• Do not sing what you hear in your headphones.

• Have a towel with you. Always!

• Do not throw the weights on the floor. Never!

• Be quiet. Quiet!

• Leave space for people to exercise around you. But don't go out of the gym!

SO WHY CAN YOU NOT GAIN WEIGHT?

What matters is the goal.

What is your real goal?

What do you want to have at the end of our workouts?

This is a program to acquire muscle mass through compound movements and accessories.

With more focus on Compounds.

1. YOU ARE NOT EATING ENOUGH. This means that you do not get the necessary calories you need every day to keep up and gain some weight in time. Ideally, you should gain 1 to 3 kilos a month. And not 1 to 3 kilos a week. At this stage you will have to make an increase in total weight and gain good muscle weight as well as fat. Fat is inevitable during a bulk diet, and it's a necessary element of our organism because it provides us with energy and is also a temperature regulator in our body. So don't worry if you see your fat percentage rise by 2%-6% or if it remains the same. Everything goes according to plan!

2. YOU ARE NOT DISCIPLINED. And by that, I mean both in your diet and your training. You can't eat properly and not train properly. And cannot train and not provide your body with the nutrients necessary to develop your muscles (protein, carbohydrates, fat, amino acids, vitamins, minerals, etc.). If you do not eat and train for a long period of time (the least I suggest is six phases of 12 weeks) then you will see no difference in your body, and you will continue to blame your genes and metabolism. For good or bad, nothing comes easy. And that's what makes it count when we finally get it. So, learn to be consistent

and do not quit on the first hardship. Waiting is hard but think about how many years you've been like this and how much it took to get here today. Since you decided to change, you have to discipline against time and be patient.

3. YOU DO NOT BECOME STRONGER. And what I mean is to do strength trainings and not just hypertrophy. You need strength training to increase your muscle volume. When you do strength training, your body adjusts to the weight you lift and learns that it has to become stronger every time. This way you build muscle and become stronger.

4. TOO MUCH PROTEIN. And I mean it. When you want to gain weight and consume a lot of protein in your meals, then you get the opposite from what you want to achieve. Protein is a basic macronutrient, but we should not go beyond 1.4g/kg of body weight. Protein makes us feel satiated, and we cannot eat as much we need to gain weight and strength. Be careful of how much you consume according to your goal. Protein does good but we need to be aware of how much and when. On the other hand, you have to increase your carbohydrates to 65% of your diet. For example, 300-350 grams. in your entire diet. Sometimes even more. What I did in my diet was the following:

carbohydrates: 420g

protein: 150g

fat: 90g

You have to learn how your body reacts to every change you make and learn to "listen" to it because there is no recipe for everyone in the world. Otherwise, we would have solved all of our problems worldwide.

5. YOU DO NOT TRAIN INTENSELY ENOUGH.

Which means how many times you train a week. To train 3 times per week is ideal if you want to maintain your weight. But if you do not train every muscle group twice every week, then you won't gain muscle volume. At least sooner than you think.

And the last and most important is

6. NOT ENOUGH PROTEIN. And this I know is contrary to what I was saying above but I wanted to state the following:

You should not eat less protein than what your muscles need for their proper replenishment and development every day.

This means that your protein in a maintenance state should range from 1.2 to 1.4g/kg of body weight.

I hope all of this helped you and added some important information about your workout and training.

So, let's see what training is and what is working out in your gym or at home!

Below are some ideas for what you can eat before training:

1 to 2 hours pre-workout:

- Protein powder with water or milk with a banana and some strawberries - all in the mixer.

- whole grain cereal with milk

- oatmeal with skim milk and a banana or some almonds

2 hours pre-workout:

- Omelet with vegetables or fruit

- Caesar salad without sauce, with a cup of rice

- less than one hour before:

- Protein bar

- 1-3 Fruits with some nuts

- Yoghurt with fruits

- Fruits with almonds

And perhaps the most important of all for just before training:

<u>5g creatine</u>

(a full tablespoon)

<u>ENERGY SOURCES WHEN WE ARE RESTING</u>

REST	FATS	GLUCOZE
FASTING	70%	30%
AFTER A MEAL	20%	80%

<u>ENERGY SOURCES WHEN TRAINING</u>

TRAINING	FATS	GLUCOZE
LOW INTENSITY	80%	20%
MEDIUM INTENSITY	50%	50%
HIGH INTENSITY	20%	80%

An hour after your workout it is very important to have a meal or take a supplement with protein and carbohydrates to replenish energy faster.

A good percentage for the post-training meal is as follows:

• Carbohydrates 70% &

• Protein 30%

To achieve better protein synthesis, the meal should be within
one hour after training.

This meal is one of the most important because it helps us to re-
pair the injured muscles during training and helps us to be
stronger in the next few days in our own or similar training.

CHAPTER THREE

BASIC METABOLIC RATE

INTRODUCTION TO YOUR DAILY AND TOTAL CALORIES

The total amount of energy (calories) needed by the body for all its vital functions in a resting state (contraction of the heart, breathing, hormone secretion, nervous system activity, etc.) is called ***Basic Metabolic Rate***.

Below is a table of decreasing or increasing daily calories that will help you a lot in your goals.

Body weight (kg) multiplied by A or B or C or D

A. 24,8	0-2 TRAININGS/WEEK
B. 26,4	1-3 TRAININGS/WEEK
C. 28,6	3-5 TRAININGS/WEEK
D. 30,8	6+ TRAININGS/WEEK

Result multiplied by 1 or 2 or 3 or 4

1. MINIMAL MOBILITY: $1.1 + 200$

2. LOW MOBILITY: $1.275 + 300$

3. MODERATE MOBILITY: $1.350 + 400$

4. HIGH MOBILITY: $1.750 + 500$

FOR BODY WEIGHT INCREASE:

In our total we add 200 or 300 calories if we have very low or low mobility accordingly.

Or add 400 or up to 550 calories if we have moderate or high mobility respectively.

We also round up the amount.

FOR BODY WEIGHT DECREASE:

Do as above but subtract the corresponding calories.

FOR BODY WEIGHT MAINTENANCE:

We do the calculations, but we do not subtract or add calories to the total.

For example, for a 30-year-old man who weighs 56 kilos, has very low mobility and wants to gain weight then the equation is as follows:

56 * 26.4 = 1478.4 * 1.1 = 1626.24 + 200 = 1826.24. And with rounding we have 1850 or 1900 calories a day. That is, if he wants to gain weight in moderation.

If you add 500 calories to this example probably you're going to end a fat trainee at the end of your workouts. Moderation is Key.

Do not forget that you have to walk at least 10,000 steps every day. That way, you are always active. Also, at the weight gain stage you have to remember to do Cardio twice a week. No more, because you will make the process harder and you will see no difference in your weight.

Weight training burns fat because you train many muscle fibres at once. You do 8 or 10 or 12 reps for 45 seconds and then sit for 90 seconds. That way you activate your body, then let it relax and then the same. So, your body uses both aerobic and anaerobic at the same time and you burn more fat.

Therefore, do not worry about your Cardio. You already do it with the weights you lift on your trainings.

And remember that what seems logical to you from outside the gym as to what to do to lose fat and to get muscle weight is exactly the opposite of what you have to do most of the times.

Our body operates very differently from our common sense. It is like the myth of losing fat in the abdomen by doing 300 ab exercises a day and continue with the same diet as before, your abs will magically appear. And yet... NO.

For your abs to show, you have to exercise them properly (with progressive overload and strength training) but you have to have a good nutrition plan. And not to forget, you have to do compound movements and include strength training in your program.

Compound movements make our waist handle more weight in time so it also builds the strength of the abdomen.

NOTHING GOOD COMES EASY.

So, if your goal is to lose weight you have to do the following:

Cardio 3%

HIIT 7%

Training with weights (Resistance training) 20%

Nutrition 70%

But if your goal is to gain weight, then you must do the following:

Cardio 1%

HIIT 2%

Training with weights (Resistance training) 47%

Nutrition 50%

TOTAL DAILY ENERGY EXPENDITURE

To calculate the details of your diet and your body rates, we must first make some calculations. Such as your total daily energy expenditure. There is a great website where you can calculate it very quickly and know how many grams per macronutrients (protein, carbs, fat) you have to consume daily if you want to gain, lose or maintain your muscle mas! Here is the site:

https://www.tdeecalculator.net

From here you can begin. It will ask you to put in your age, your weight, your height, your approximate fat percentage, and the number of trainings per week.

If this training program you will follow with us is your first and you hit the gym 2-3 times a week in average, then put in 3-5 times a week.

Then scroll down to "bulking" and take a look at the tabs. You will choose the one that says "high carb". With those percentages you can go to a dietician and give the exact information you want to get a diet that fits you exactly.

Below is a typical dietary day that I go through during my winter training.

It's not much as far as cooking and preparation, because it contains fruit and nuts, cottage and some meals I can have with me in a lunch box at work.

BREAKFAST	300g MILK	100g OAK & CEREAL	
INTERMEDIATE	200g FRUIT & 23 ALMONDS	or Shake Protein & Fruit	
NOON	400g. BLACK PEAS	200gr. MEATBALL OR 200gr. FISH	ONE SLICE SANDWICH BREAD
TRAINING	WEIGHTS & AEROBIC	500-700kcal	
POST-TRAINING MEAL	200gr. FRUIT & 23 ALMONDS	or Shake Protein & Fruit.	
INTERMEDIATE	1 CUP OF COTTAGE		
AFTERNOON	200gr. FRUIT & 23 ALMONDS		
DINNER	150g BLACK PEAS	200g MEATBALL OR 200g FISH	ONE SLICE SANDWICH BREAD

But let's just go over to the main issue, which is Macronutrients.

Total:

1. carbohydrates - 409g

2. protein - 245g

3. fat - 72g

Total calories = 3350kcal

In general, try to note down the calories you consume every day in your meals. You can get help on that from several apps on your smartphone where you can add whatever you eat or even scan the labels of the product and you get exactly the calories and the ingredients you consume.

Another option I would suggest, is to ask from your nutrition-ist a detailed day-by-day program according to the calories you wish to consume every day.

Chapter Four

The Content of Training

THE BOOK CONTAINS 12 WEEKS DIVIDED AS
FOLLOWS:

1. THE FIRST 2 WEEKS IS STRENGTH WHICH MEANS
THAT WE PUT ON EXTRA WEIGHTS FOR FEWER REPS.
IN PARTICULAR, 6 REPS.

This way, you learn how much you can lift and with an app that
calculates your strength percentages per unit of weight you can
calculate every week how many kilos you put on for each exercise. An easy way to calculate them is through this website:

https://tinyurl.com/ydcx7ukf

or full direct address:

https://exrx.net/Calculators/OneRepMax

So, after completing the first two weeks and becoming stronger
and have noted how many kilos you have put in in each exercise,
then it's time to insert on this website how much you lifted to get
your percentages. Strength trainings are a big benefit to the
whole of our training as they help our body become stronger as
well as gain bulk. In strength training we want explosiveness.

Our eccentric is slow (3 to 4 seconds) and the concentric is fast (1 to 2 seconds) as we move the weights up and shorten the muscles.. This way we combine both types of muscle fibers into our body. Type I and type II, or slow and fast.

2. THE NEXT 3 WEEKS ARE HYPERTROPHY. MEANING THAT WE WILL USE THE PROTOCOL OF 4 SETS OF 10 REPS.

These reps are used when we want to gain muscle volume, that is, to obtain muscle hypertrophy. It's that 'PUMP' we feel after training. Our muscles fill with blood and lactic acid and are more hydrated. That way they get that 'pump' and after training with good and nutritious food and good rest (7 to 9 hours) hypertrophy becomes reality. During these weeks, we will emphasise how we carry the weights up and down. The concentric contraction should be 2 seconds, then pause for a second when we are up and the eccentric contraction should be 3 or 4 seconds and then immediately up again (concentric) in 1-2 seconds.

This way we keep the muscle in continuous bending and stretching for a longer period of time and we assist the operation of hypertrophy. In substance, we destroy more muscle fibres so our body can adjust and create more for the next time. It's like causing a shock to our body every time and helping it get better in every training.

3. THE NEXT TWO WEEKS ARE STRENGTH AGAIN AND THE FOLLOWING TWO HYPERTROPHY AGAIN SO THAT WE REACH THE 10TH WEEK WHICH IS A LARGE CHALLENGE.

It's like a powerlifting contest with 5 workouts per week in 2 compound movements per day and one abdominal exercise. This prepares us for the final 2 weeks.

4. THE LAST 2 WEEKS ARE HYPERTROPHY IN THE MODEL OF 6 SETS AND 10 REPS.

There are 6 workouts per week and rest day can be either at the end of the week or between the 3 workouts. These last two weeks are certainly harder and more challenging, but they are the ones that will determine if you really want to make a good change to your body. Remember, however, that through these twelve weeks you won't have the exact body of your dreams, but you will have laid a very solid foundation to build the body of your dreams in the months to follow. For this reason, stay tuned to our page on Instagram for the next books and exercises we will upload to help your body, yourself and also your spirit to head for something better than what you have now. It is important to learn to exercise better, but also to know where all these exercises and protocols benefit each time. Do not follow blindly what is suggested to you.

SO WHY DO A HYPERTROPHY PROGRAM?

* Because if it's winter you can eat more in relation to summer.

* Because you are tired of being weak and want to see a serious change in your body.

* Because you like to eat a lot and now it's time to put on some muscle weight and lose some fat.

* Because with the exercises we will do in our workouts you will learn your body better and your daily life will become much better.

* Because you will learn to eat and think properly inside and outside the gym.

- To learn how hypertrophy training works and to love being free of clothes.

- Because we all want to double in volume and not only in size, but we don't know how to do it properly.

- Because bodybuilding trainings help you build the body's aesthetic and better understand your body.

- Because with these trainings you will have a greater variety in exercises compared to other training models such as power-lifting, Olympic lifting, strongman. The exercises that take place in such sports are specific and as time passes, you do the same exercises with more weight and more times a week. The reps do not change, the set may change, and the resting time does not change (it's almost always 3 to 5 minutes so your neuromuscular system can better replenish the weights you lifted and be ready for the next repeat).

- Because with these trainings you will feel better at the end of each Phase. You will look forward to the next Phase and have your new exercises and your new results. Our training program consists of 6 Phases shaped so that you get the best results in your body.

So, we have included in our program an extra two weeks. One is a powerlifting contest. In that week, you will have many sets of 2 reps in basic compound exercises. This will help you understand how much you've grown in relation to your first week of checking and noting how many kilos you can lift. And the second extra week is at the end of the training and is called deload week. This week you can practice from 1 to 3 sessions a week just to keep in shape.

Also, any muscle imbalances you may have in your body, such as your biceps (right or left), either in your legs or arms, you can correct, so both look the same. You cannot change how the muscle fibres are formed inside your body, but you can change a different looking arm or leg. You can do that by always begin with your weaker part first. After you finish the SET you perform another 4-5 reps with the imbalanced muscle. That way you help your muscle to grow and look like the other one. It will take time and effort. Don't wait immediate results.

In short, we created this book so you can train to develop your muscle mass. However, with the right nutrition, you can also just maintain your weight. The recipe is simple:

• add 4 to 5 times Cardio instead of 2 to the existing program.

• Focus more on your nutrition, which means taking more protein to your whole macronutrients at 2.0g to 2.4g/kg per kilo of bodyweight. For pounds divide the total by 2.2.

• R E L A X. Do your workouts, keep the right nutrition and everything will be fine.

• Remember to be consistent in your training and nutrition.

• Be patient because nothing good comes easy. Nothing is done fast. And everything that does, it is dissolved even faster.

• Be strong and smile every day. In essence, from here on that's how you'll be. Exercising elevates the levels of testosterone, the growth hormone and endorphins and because of that you are happier and more active in your day.

• Learn to be consistent and true to your goals, otherwise you will not see the results you expect. An average waiting time is 6 months. 6 months of good workouts, balanced nutrition and good rest is equivalent to many beautiful effects on your body and spirit.

• Always log the weights you lift. We have created a separate cell next to set and reps so you can log the kilos/pounds you lift for each exercise. The best would be to note how much you lifted on the first set and how much on the last one. It is very important to note your weights so that your help yourself do a proper progressive overload in weights every week. This is achieved with a 2.5% added weight per week per exercise. So don't forget to note down your kilos on the form we have created.

• Sleep for 7 to 9 hours. We have said this many times and we will keep saying it. Because sleep is the biggest anabolic in hypertrophy. Insufficient levels of sleep mean our body does not get the chance to make up for the injured cells that were lost during the training and the next day we will not have progressed as much as we should. Be consistent. Once more. Be consistent. Think of your future self. That way, you will be able to move forward, even when you want to stay in your house.

• Stretch before and after. Dynamic stretching before training that mimic the movements of the exercises you will do without or with light weights. Also, static stretching at the end of the trainings for better muscle recovery over the next few days. Below we have included some stretches with illustrations and explanations.

• Watch videos, read articles from us and from other pages and be informed on what you're doing. Always have a more general image of the things you occupy yourself with. It's good for your workouts, but more importantly for yourself.

Remember that CARDIO is important but in the right way.

This mentality of endless hours on the treadmill, circuit programs and high-intensity training with minimal breaks was a sort of marketing from a bygone era that never seems to go away.

You have to understand that Cardio helps you lose fat while you're doing it. And it does not need to be in great intensity. Moderate-intensity walking with a low or high incline (depending on how much your knees can take) is enough to do the job.

On the other hand, resistance training (weight training) make the body burn fat while not in the gym. In short terms, that is.

The compound exercises (squats, deadlifts, hip thrusts, chest presses, shoulder presses, rowing, etc.) use a lot of muscles in our body and in this way, more muscles stay on alert and the body learns to be on alert until the next training.

And that's why we burn fat while we're out of the gym.

Chapter Five

Who we are
A Few Words About Us

All this started when one day we simply wanted to change the way we see our body and ourselves in general. So, we decided to start reading and working out. One started to help the other and steadily we started to get the results we were expecting. But unfortunately, not in the time, nor the way we wanted. We waited for everything to magically appear and eventually, with good training and nutrition (also sweets and junk food from time to time) make the big change. But those things do not change as fast as we expect them to. The thing is that the time it took to make the change and start fitness and nutrition, was the same as to see the changes. Because unfortunately we did not know then how to do it and had do it by ourselves. Find the right exercises, read thousands of articles on nutrition, fitness, relaxation, supplements, (mind-muscle connection - a concept to be discussed below).

In general, it was a time-consuming process that took on for years, without us realizing. We could perhaps have evaded some if we let gave up on our selfishness and shame and just decided to ask others or at least start professional training. For us at least, our careers in the field of fitness and nutrition started as amateurs.

So, since we started making mistakes, we learned things about ourselves, we asked, learned, tried in our way, tried in other ways, watched videos, attended seminars for personal & weight training, heard tips from renowned teachers and coaches for training and nutrition and we arrived at the point where we want to pass it all on to the rest of the world. But with one extra detail. To change the way we think.

Unless we change the way we think about fitness and nutrition, we will not change our way of life. It is a change that has to be done properly and in coordination with our Health. We need to connect the mind and body in this change otherwise there will be no CHANGE. If we do not properly synchronize our minds and body we are not going to move forward. And if indeed we do, they will be wrong steps and we will have to start from the beginning. If we aim for the beach, a relationship, a photo or something that fills the void in our vanity then we have set full sail towards failure. Good or bad, that's the truth and that's where those who follow vanity and not the path of their health, mental and physical, end up.

It is therefore important for us to set some conditions and to lay the foundations for a long-term relationship between fitness and nutrition. We do not want something temporary or topical. We want something that lasts in time.

What you need is patience, will, discipline, vision and persistence towards these goals. It's something that will stay with you for many years and it's something you have to think of as fun and enjoyable. If you do just for the sake of doing it then there's no meaning. Fitness and nutrition are two essential elements to well-being. It's the first step so that we are strong and tough in the face of everything that arises in our lives. Because the discipline and the vision we have through our trainings make us set goals and not give up of a whim. While our patience makes us stronger and more adaptable to anything that at us and tries to change our course.

On the other hand, our will and persistence make us want to believe more in these goals and not to give up on what we love to do in our lives.

So, we came to our conclusion about exercising and proper nutrition. It is a mindset and a joyful way of life. It helps us respond better to difficult situations, but it is also the fuel that pushes us to carry on when we believe that everything has been lost.

All we want to accomplish and expect to feel in order to begin every journey in our life is within us. And if we take a good look inside, we will find everything we seek around us and we will accomplish all we believe we do not deserve.

Because we have but one life and have to live it in all its greatness.

We wish you enjoy the way we write and decode exercising and nutrition through the 12 labors of Hercules.

HOW DID I BEGIN? A SMALL STORY

8 years ago, I started going to the gym. I started then with a good friend who was involved in competitive martial arts and had seen something good in me and the discipline I have for other things like music (piano, bass and guitar).

I was a very different person, however. I was smoking a lot during the day, I was going out often, drinking, did not sleep well (usually I was sleeping in the morning) but thankfully I was walking a lot. So, I started going to the gym and I remember my friend's advice for eating well after we finish our training. So, we would finish training and go to eat. Afterwards I would of course light my cigarette to supplement my micronutrients!

So it went on, slowly, until the call came for my military service and all these things were now in the past. I enlisted in the army and suddenly I raised a shed in front of me. Big one, mind you. I gained 14 kilos while in the military. And it was surely not muscles!

I always thought, though, that I like to work out and as long as I was in the army I was trying to do so in a small gym we had, 1 to 2 times a week.

On the other hand, I was thinking about my bad nutrition, my heavy smoking, and not taking care of myself.

When I finished my service and returned to the real world, I decided to start a diet. I was at my lowest point.

So, I started dieting 3 days before the Easter good week, a week when everyone was eating mountains and me, 100g of meat, 100g of rice and salad.

I endured because I wanted to prove to myself that I can and deserve to be better than before! And I did it. I lost 16 kilos in 4 months.

After Easter was over and I returned home I registered to a gym. I did an hour of weight training, and in the afternoon, I did an hour of cycling. I never remember myself taking more than an hour at the gym. In very rare cases I took one and a half hours only when I was practising on strength training.

Since then, I got somewhat better in my endurance and body and I began to enjoy the whole process.

I was doing quite well but I was very concerned about the fact that I was smoking a lot and then, as time went by and I thought about it more, I was smoking even more for some reason.

A great advantage was that I was reading a lot. Books on leadership, marketing, positive thinking, psychology, abundance and self-presentation. So, since I had written my goals down and read them every day, I decided to do the same for my smoking issue.

After I managed to quit for good a little over a year ago, I sat and wrote down why I don't want to do it and some reasons that I must not for the people I love. And I was reading them every day. Every time I remembered it, I was reading it.

Here is what I wrote:

"Smoking is harmful to my health

I've quit smoking.

I have quit smoking because it's harmful to me and the people I love.

I have quit smoking for a better present and future together with the people I love.

Cigarette is completely gone from of my life because it is harmful to my health.

I have quit smoking because it is harmful to my health.

Everything that is harmful and destructive to me and the people I love, I will remove from my life.

That's why I've quit smoking, because it's bad for my health.

Everything that is harmful and destructive to me and the people I love, I will remove from my life. Smoking is harmful to my health.

Everything that is harmful and destructive to me and the people I love, I will remove from my life.

I desire everything that is positive, constructive, healthy and better for me and the people I love."

I read this passage over, and over, and over again until a few months later, it stuck to my subconscious. I saw in my sleep that I was smoking and was so saddened that I had put such an effort to quit only to start again, and when I woke up, I felt so relieved and happy that it was just a dream. From then on, I knew that whatever I want to do in my life, I can make it. Because smoking is something so subconsciously rooted within by years of addiction, that it's hard to give up.

It was indeed like that. Since then, I succeeded in every goal I set.

I stopped sugar 3 months ago, I've been off white flour for a month, refreshments for a year, ice cream (to which all of us are addicted) for a while and whatever I wanted to cut or challenge myself, I did. The more we do for ourselves and we say no to bad habits, the easier it is to make it in the future.

Of what I learned, one is certain. There is no partial fulfilment of the goal. I reduced cigarettes to 5 a day. But I suffered a lot. I was looking forward to the next cigarette with my eyes on the clock. The best way is to quit your habit immediately and find something else to replace it with.

So, one day after training I analyzed how many hours I spent on cigarettes. About 5 hours, since I had about 30 cigarettes a day. So, I put on another hour of cycling, another hour of reading, another hour of walking and slept a lot to not think about it. And I did it. Until this day, as I'm writing this book, I have not smoked at all.

Since then, I said that I will get used to a good way of life, working out, nutrition, sleeping and everything else I know, I will try to teach to the people around me.

Because knowledge not shared is knowledge lost.

So, during the last few years I have been occupied with working out more professionally, completing a great course in a school for personal training. From the school I acquired many important things, first for me and secondly for the people who so desperately wanted my help.

Because I like to learn, to read, to experiment, I wanted to do this right. Not train someone without knowing how and why. And I did it. Because when you become very good at what you do, ultimately others believe in you because they see in you what they want and to get it they ask you how. It matters not what you are, but who you are and why you do it so well!

Our character is our future, said Heraclitus once and he was absolutely right. The best coach in the world with the worst attitude will never become his best self. Simple as that.

That is why we must grow both our body and our mind. It is a journey of multiple processes. We need to know why we work out. We need to know how to eat. But first of all, we must know ourselves.

Everything starts from us. No one is waiting for us to begin. We have to take the first steps towards change to change something radically. Nothing comes easy and that's why it deserves more in the end.

But gymnastics and knowledge never end. You do not exercise to stop doing so at some point or to stop learning and reading. You work out to have energy for your day-to-day activities and you read to become better at everything you do daily and whatever fills you up.

Things are simple, we just tend to make them difficult using a bunch of excuses and tricks to not exercise, not walk, not read a good book, not leave home and the comfortable couch.

But when we leave exercising to the next day, we have to re-member that sometime our health will leave us for the next day. And then it will be late.

We need slow and steady steps towards our goal.

There is no quick solution. And whoever says he found it, he has found the solution to disaster.

Magic pills and special belts for losing fat do not exist. There exist only gullible people who are afraid they will not make it in their lives.

Remember that we have but one life and we must live it dynami-cally and uniquely. To it greatness. A second one we will never have!

From here on, your own journey begins, and we must now put in order all that you will learn in this book with the labors of Hercules.

Whether you're a boy or a girl, a man or a woman, this book will teach you how to become a better person. No matter race, religion or nationality.

This book refers to people who want to become better and to offer something better to our planet.

Because only like this our planet become better, along with every person living on it.

And remember this:

"The best Coach in the world for your success in any field is the Mind."

Chapter Six

Introduction to Stretching
Dynamic and Static

Dynamic stretches are intended to warm up the muscles we are about to train to help our body respond better to the training. To avoid lack or range of motion and injuries during training.

Always remember to perform dynamic stretches before your trainings and at the end of them, do static stretches from 20" to 30" at each stretch for the exact same reason.

Stretches must be performed slowly and steadily to the point that we don't feel the muscle being stretched intensely. Otherwise, we get the opposite effect from stretching.

We provide you with pre-training (dynamic) and post-training stretches (static).

Let's begin!

DYNAMIC STRETCHING

UPPER BODY:

- Shoulder Circles

- Internal (for Pecs and Biceps) or External (for Lats and Rear Delts) Rotation depending on your workout

- Cat and Cow

- rear belts w/ band

- or mimic the motion of the exercises you are going to perform with lower weights.

LOWER BODY:

- Squat and hold for 20 seconds

- Bodyweight Split squat

- Leg swings back and forth or side to side

- Butterfly with movement

- Bodyweight Standing Calves

STATIC STRETCHING

LOWER BODY:

- Inner thigh stretch (butterfly)
- Hip Flexor Lunge Stretch
- Hamstrings Stretch
- Calves
- Standing Quad Stretch
- Glute Stretch
- IT Band Stretch

UPPER BODY:

- Neck Stretch
- Overhead Triceps Stretch
- Cross-body shoulder stretch
- Biceps Stretch
- Chest Stretch
- Standing wall Stretch
- Thread the Needle Stretch
- Wrist Extension and Flexion Stretch
- Child's Pose Stretch

THE LABORS OF HERCULES

The Twelve Labors of Hercules are a very good comparison to the struggles we've gone through in our lives. Training is a term different from exercising. Training involves a Goal (Bulk or Cut) and a Plan (strength exercises, hypertrophy exercises, endurance exercises etc.).

While exercising means that you are in an athletic facility (gym) and just do a series of exercises that you have chosen randomly each time and just maintain your physical condition.

The Twelve Labors of Hercules have to do with you training right and learning of the exercises through repetition and correct attitude of the trainee through the trainings. It is important that you learn to exercise properly.

With the right exercise technique, the right breaks between sets and the correct nutrition through the rest of the day.

All are essential to a training and for that reason we must make sure that your training and the way you think during it, is correct. Nothing is left to chance because everything has a small effect overall Goal.

So, keep your mind clear, your thoughts aimed at the Goal, and everything will go as planned.

THE TWELVE LABORS OF HERCULES

Hercules' Labors have been recorded in Greek mythology as twelve accomplishments done by the mythical hero Hercules, in order to cleanse himself for the murder of his wife and his children, which he committed when Hera drove him mad. For this purpose, Hercules went to the Oracle of Delphi and received a prophecy, according to which he had to serve Eurystheus, king of Tiryns for twelve years, and to perform the labors that he was ordering. The labors he eventually did were:

1. His first feat was the extermination of the terrible lion of Nemea, which had desolated the whole state.

2. His second accomplishment was the extermination of Lernaean Hydra, a nine-headed monster who lived on Lerni lake and spread disaster to the locals. In the place of every head that was cut by Hercules, two more thrusted out, and so he was forced burn the neck of each head he cut. Then, after he had killed the beast, he dipped his arrows into its blood and made them deadly.

3. The third feat was where he caught the deer of Kyrenia with the bronze legs and golden horns and brought to Eurystheus alive.

4. Fourth, he killed the boar of Erymanthus, that brought panic and desolation to Arcadia.

5. Fifth, he cleaned the stables of Augeas, the rich king with 3,000 oxen, from the manure that had piled on for thirty years, the last time the stables were cleaned. Hercules cleaned them by diverting the waters of Penius and Alphaeus toward the stables, which washed out the manure.

6. Sixth, he killed the Stymphalian Birds with his arrows, which were man-eating birds with bronze beaks, nails and wings, and flew like shuttles.

7. Seventh, he grabbed the wild bull of Crete, which caused destruction on all of Crete, and took it alive to Eurystheus, who was frightened and set him free.

8. Hercules' eighth feat was the rapture of Diomedes' wild horses. He was the king of Vistons in Thrace, son of Mars, who was feeding his wild horses with human meat. Diomidis was killed by Hercules and, taking his horses, he went to Eurystheus after he had tamed them. The King of Mycenae set them free in Mount Olympus, where they were devoured by wild beasts.

9. Following this achievement of Hercules, Euristhea's daughter, Admite, asked to bring her the belt of Hippolyte, the queen of the Amazons, and Eurystheus ordered Hercules to fulfill his daughter's desire. Hercules, after many adventures, found the Amazon warrior people and tried to take their queen's life. But they fought him so wildly and so fiercely refused to give him what he wanted, so that Heracles was forced to kill Hippolyte and take the belt.

10. Then Eurystheus ordered him to fetch him the oxen of Geryon, which were guarded by Orthros, a terrible dog. Geryon was a giant with three bodies and three heads who lived on an island on the western edge of the Ocean. After many struggles and after fighting the waves to reach the island, he killed Geryon and his dog Orthros. This was his tenth achievement.

11. His eleventh feat was the harvesting of the apples of Hesperides. The Hesperides were nymphs who lived in the garden of gods, tasked to guard the golden apples that were there, gifted by Gaia in the wedding of Zeus and Hera.

Along with these daughters of the Night, guardian of the garden stood the terrible Dragon Ladon, as well as Atlas who held up the sky. The gods' garden was on the westernmost borders of the earth, where the sky and earth met on an island beyond the ocean or near Libya, in an African mountain. Hercules took the apples with the help of Atlas, taking the weight of the sky on his shoulders for a bit until Atlas stole the apples from the Garden of the Hesperides.

12. Finally, Hercules' twelfth feat was to descend to Hades and to bring to the surface and to Eurystheus the three-eyed dog, Cerverus, who was the son of Typhon and Echinda, his brothers the two-headed Orthros, the dog of Geryon, and the Lernaean Hydra and guarded the gates of the Underworld.

Hercules, with these twelve accomplishments, was freed from the rule of Eurystheus and then roamed the world helping the weak (Source: https://en.wikipedia.org/wiki/Labours_of_Hercules).

Below is the pentathlon, its sports, but also what they represent to the human as a whole! Because in Ancient Greece, nothing was by chance. Everything was done for some ultimate goal!

1. BODY - ROAD

2. SOUL - FIGHT

3. SPIRIT - JUMP

4. BRAIN - DISC

5. THOUGHT - SPEAR

The best we can do as humans is to evolve as a whole and not partially. There are many examples of people who only had a beautiful body but no mind to respond to their financial variations. Or they did not have the morality (soul) to keep the balance.

Educated people who did not care for their health altogether, they did not walk, nor did they eat properly. People who made millions but have not looked after their body or mind, nor their soul and in the end, they either lost it all, or ruined their health or when they left this world, they were not remembered by anyone for something good. Or even nothing at all.

It is very important, therefore, to grow every aspect of ourselves as a whole and not partially. We should exercise and mind our diet, but still the most important thing is to mind what our brain and our soul eat every day. No one is better than the other. We need to remember that every time. To work collectively and give value to all people around us. To hang out with those who change us for the better, who are positive and constructive people.

For this reason, you should know yourself well, learn how react to change and learn how to become better. Always think of how to teach what you know to others because knowledge not shared, is useless. And remember that when we let others speak, we can always learn something new. Because we never learn anything new from what we say to others. We have one mouth but two ears! so as to listen more (knowledge) and speak less.

Let your actions speak for themselves, not your mouth. People appreciated that more.

Below are twenty (20) of the DOLPHICAL ORDERS:

1. Become a philosopher – ΦΙΛΟΣΟΦΟΣ ΓΙΝΟΥ

2. Seek Wisdom – ΣΟΦΙΑ ΖΗΤΕΙ

3. Know Yourself – ΓΝΩΘΙ ΣΑΥΤΟΝ

4. Dominate yourself – ΑΡΧΕ ΣΕΑΥΤΟΥ

5. Communicate with the wise – ΣΟΦΟΙΣ ΧΡΩ

6. Everything in moderation – ΜΕΤΡΟΝ ΑΡΙΣΤΟΝ

7. Nothing in excess – ΜΗΔΕΝ ΑΓΑΝ

8. Do not blame anyone – ΨΕΓΕ ΜΗΔΕΝΑ

9. Speak good for all – ΕΥΛΟΓΕΙ ΠΑΝΤΑΣ

10. Do not waste your time – ΧΡΟΝΟ ΦΕΙΔΟΥ

11. Striking a righteous right – ΠΟΝΕΙ ΜΕΤΑ ΔΙΚΑΙΟΥ

12. Control your tongue - ΓΛΩΤΤΗΣ ΑΡΧΗ

13. Dissolve animosities – ΕΧΘΡΑΣ ΔΙΑΛΥΕ

14. Do not take pride on your strength – ΕΠΙ ΡΩΜΗ ΜΗ ΚΑΥΧΩ

15. Respect yourself – ΣΕΑΥΤΟΝ ΑΙΔΟΥ

16. Consider what is useful- ΒΟΛΕΥΟΥ ΧΡΗΣΙΜΑ

17. When you have, give – ΕΧΩΝ ΧΑΡΙΖΟΥ

18. Do not believe in luck – ΤΥΧΗ ΜΗ ΠΙΣΤΕΥΕ

19. Fight for justice – ΗΤΤΩ ΥΠΕΡ ΔΙΚΑΙΟΥ

20. Die without sadness – ΤΕΛΕΥΤΑ ΑΛΥΠΟΣ

Use them in your life, your daily routine, your workouts, your relationships, and you will see how your life will change for the better.

The ancient Greeks understood the meaning of well-being and the right mentality thousands of years before, and we must learn to apply them to our lives for better results.

Also remember that everything takes time and patience to complete. Do not be impatient and take the wrong steps.

You will be taken more steps back and will have to make more effort to get back in the position you were.

Be Focused, Strong and Consistent.

"It is incredible, the effect of small and steady steps in the final result with the passing of time"

Robin Sharma

CHAPTER SEVEN

THE TRAINING OF HERCULES

IT IS TIME TO BECOME THE BEST VERSION OF YOUR SELF

The time we all have been waiting for has come.
To make trainings a reality in order to prepare for the twelve labors of HERCULES.

To be able to change yourself and your body for good. Now it's time to become stronger and see your body reach new levels of strength and hypertrophy. Start Hercules' program and fear nothing, because the twelve gods of Olympus are with you and they protect you in every Phase.

In our Instagram page we have included a pre-training video with dynamic stretches as well as pre-training static stretches to help you recover after training.

Stay focused, strong and tuned in on our page at the end of this book.

STRENGTH - WEEK 1 & 2

VOLUME 75% - 85% 1RM

REST: 3 '- 5'

FREQUENCY 4X/Week

10 MINUTES DYNAMIC STRETCHES BEFORE TRAINING

AND 10 MINUTES STATIC AFTER TRAINING.

DAY ONE: LOWER	SETS * REPS	WEIGHT / EXERCISE:
BACK SQUAT	3*6	
LEG EXT.	3*6	
INCLINE PRESS	3*6	
LANDMINE PRESS	3*6	
PUSH PRESS	3*6	
PLANK	4*45sec	
SEATED CALF RAISE	4*15	

DAY TWO: UPPER	SETS * REPS	WEIGHT / EXERCISE
RACK PULL	3*6	
PULL UPS (WEIGHTED)	3*6	
T-BAR	3*6	
SHRUGS (wide grip)	3*6	
CLOSE GRIP PRESS	3*6	
LEG RAISES	4*15	
SEATED CALF RAISE	4*15	

DAY THREE: LOWER/ DELTS	SETS * REPS	WEIGHT / EXERCISE
RDL'S	3*6	
GLUTE BRIDGE	3*6	
LEG PRESS	3*6	
HAM CURLS	3*6	
BB HIGH PULL	3*6	
ACCORDION CRUNCHES	4*20	
SEATED CALF RAISE	4*15	

DAY FOUR: UPPER/ LOWER	SETS * REPS	WEIGHT / EXERCISE
CHEST PRESS	3*6	
DIPS	3*6	
PULL UPS	3*6	
BENTOVER ROWS	3*6	
REAR DELTS (DB)	3*6	
ACCORDION CRUNCHES	4*20	
SEATED CALF RAISE	4*15	

HYPERTROPHY - WEEK 3 & 4

VOLUME 75% 1RM

REST 90" - 120"

FREQUENCY: 5x/Week

10 MINUTES DYNAMIC STRETCHES BEFORE TRAINING

AND 10 MINUTES STATIC AFTER TRAINING.

DAY ONE: PUSH	SETS * REPS	WEIGHT / EXERCISE
CHEST PRESS (BB)	4*10	
DIPS	4*10	
INCLINE FLYS (30° +45°)	4*10	
CROSSOVER (mid pulley)	4*10	
SKULL CRUSHERS	4*10	
CABLE EXT.	4*10	
HANGING OBLIQUES	4*12	
RUSSIAN TWISTS	4*12	

DAY TWO: PULL	SETS * REPS	WEIGHT / EXERCISE
ROWS	4*10	
PULL UP	4*10	
T-BAR	4*10	
UPRIGHT ROWS	4*10	
INCLINE BICEP CURLS (DB)	4*10	
HAMMER CURLS	4*10	
PLANK	4*45sec	

DAY THREE: LEGS	SETS * REPS	WEIGHT / EXERCISE
LEG PRESS (BASIC STANCE)	4*10	
LEG EXT. (UNILATERAL)	4*10	
BACK SQUAT	4*10	
ABDUCTION (MACHINE)	4*10	
ADDUCTION (MACHINE	4*10	
BICYCLE CRUNCHES	4*15	
STANDING CALVES	4*15	

DAY FOUR: UPPER	SETS * REPS	WEIGHT / EXERCISE
BENCH PRESS	4*10	
FRENCH PRESS (CABLE)	4*10	
DEADLIFT	4*10	
LATERAL RAISES	4*10	
MILITARY PRESS	4*10	
REVERSE CURLS	4*10	
CHIN DOWNS	4*10	

DAY FIVE: LOWER	SETS * REPS	WEIGHT / EXERCISE
RDL'S	4*10	
GLUTE BRIDGE	4*10	
HAM CURLS	4*10	
SWINGS	4*10	
BULGARIAN SPLIT SQUAT	4*10	
STANDING CALVES	4*15	
SIDE PLANK (EACH SIDE)	4*30sec	

STRENGTH - WEEK 5 & 6

VOLUME 90% 1RM

REST 210sec - 300sec

FREQUENCY: 4x/Week

10 MINUTES DYNAMIC STRETCHES BEFORE TRAINING

AND 10 MINUTES STATIC AFTER TRAINING.

On the exercises that mentions +1*2 you do first the repetitions written, then you rest for 15 seconds and you do one more plus one more after another 15 seconds rest.

DAY ONE: BACK / ABS	SETS * REPS WEIGHT / EXERCISE
DEADLIFT	4*3 +1*2
PULL UPS	4*3
CHIN UPS	4*3
T-BAR W/ V-GRIP	4*3
BARBELL CURLS	4*8
PREACHER CURLS	4*8
CABLE CRUNCHES	4*15

DAY TWO: LEGS / DELTS / ABS	SETS * REPS	WEIGHT / EXERCISE
BACK SQUAT	4*3 +1*2	
LEG EXT. (TOES OUT)	4*3	
LEG PRESS (HIGH FEET - TOES INWARDS)	4*3	
MILITARY PRESS	4*3	
UPRIGHT ROWS	4*8	
REAR DELTS (CABLE)	4*8	
PLANK (WEIGHTED)	4*45sec	

DAY THREE: CHEST / ABS	SETS * REPS	WEIGHT / EXERCISE
CHEST PRESS (BB)	4*3	
INCLINE PRESS	4*3 +1*2	
LANDMINE PRESS	4*3	
CLOSE GRIP PRESS	4*8	
ROPE EXT.	4*8	
OVERHEAD EXT.	4*8	
ROLL OUT	4*15	

DAY FOUR: LEGS / DELTS / ABS	SETS * REPS	WEIGHT / EXERCISE
GLUTE BRIDGE	4*3 +1*2	
LEG CURLS	4*3 +1*2	
RDL'S (NARROW FEET)	4*3	
PUSH PRESS	4*3	
FRONT RAISES	4*8	
BACK EXTENSIONS	4*10	
KNEELING WOOD CHOPS	4*15	

HYPERTROPHY - WEEK 7 & 8

VOLUME: 70% 1RM

REST: 90sec - 120sec

FREQUENCY: 5x/Week

10 MINUTES DYNAMIC STRETCHES BEFORE TRAINING

AND 10 MINUTES STATIC AFTER TRAINING.

DAY ONE: LEGS / ABS	SETS * REPS	WEIGHT / EXERCISE
FRONT SQUAT	5*5	
LEG PRESS (NARROW STANCE)	5*10	
WALKING LUNGES (WIDE FEET)	5*10	
SUMO DEADLIFTS	5*10	
STANDING CALVES	5*10	
LEG EXT.	5*10	
FRONT RAISES	5*10	
CABLE CRUNCHES	5*10	
WIDE PLANK (WEIGHTED)	5*40sec	

DAY TWO: BACK / CHEST / ABS	SETS * REPS	WEIGHT / EXERCISE
T-BAR ROWS	5*5	
SINGLE ARM ROW (DB)	5*10	
V-GRIP PULL DOWNS	5*10	
PULL UPS (WIDE GRIP)	5*FAIL	
CHEST PRESS (DB)	5*10	
CABLE FLYS (LOW PULLEY)	5*10	
DIPS	5*10	
SUPERMANS	5*15	

DAY THREE: LEGS / ABS	SETS * REPS	WEIGHT / EXERCISE
HIP THRUST	5*5	
DUMBBELL RDL'S	5*10	
HAMSTRING CURLS	5*10,8,8,6,4	
LEG PRESS (FEET UP)	5*10	
STANDING CALVES	5*10	
CABLE PULL THROUGHS	5*10	
LATERAL RAISES	5*10	
RUSSIAN TWISTS (WEIGHTED)	5*12	

DAY FOUR: PULL / ABS	SETS * REPS	WEIGHT / EXERCISE
LATERAL BICEP CURLS	5*10	
BICEP CURLS (DB)	5*10	
PREACHER CURLS	5*10	
STANDING WRIST CURLS	5*10	
REAR DELTS (MACHINE)	5*10	
STRAIGHT ARMS PULLDOWNS	5*10	
DEADLIFTS	5*10	
OTIS UPS (WEIGHTED)	5*10	

DAY FIVE: PUSH / ABS	SETS * REPS	WEIGHT / EXERCISE
MILITARY PRESS	5*5	
REVERSE GRIP EXT.	5*10	
CROSS BENCH DIPS	5*10	
REVERSE FRENCH PRESS	5*10	
CLOSE GRIP PRESS	5*10	
BENCH PRESS	5*10,8,8,6,4	
FLYS (FLAT BENCH)	5*10	
V-UPS	5*10	

POWERLIFTING COMPETITION

CONTEST - WEEK 9

VOLUME 95%± 1RM

REST 180sec - 300sec

FREQUENCY: 5x/Week

10 MINUTES DYNAMIC STRETCHES BEFORE TRAINING

AND 10 MINUTES STATIC AFTER TRAINING.

DAY ONE: LEGS / ABS	SETS * REPS	WEIGHT / EXERCISE
BACK SQUATS	6*6,5,4,3,2,1	
GLUTE BRIDGE	6*6,5,4,3,2,1	
PUSH PRESS	6*6,5,4,3,2,1	
LEG PRESS	6*6,5,4,3,2,1	
SEATED CALVES	6*20	
LEG RAISES	6*15	

DAY TWO: BACK / ABS	SETS * REPS	WEIGHT / EXERCISE
DEADLIFT OR RACK PULLS	6*6,5,4,3,2,1	
BENT OVER ROWS	6*6,5,4,3,2,1	
PULL UPS	6*6,5,4,3,2,1	
BARBELL CURLS	6*6,5,4,4,4,4	
OTIS UPS	5*15	

DAY THREE: CHEST / ABS	SETS * REPS	WEIGHT / EXERCISE
CHEST PRESS	6*6,5,4,3,2,1	
DIPS	6*6,5,4,3,2,2	
MILITARY PRESS	6*6,5,4,3,2,1	
INCLINE PRESS	6*6,5,4,3,2,1	
SEATED CALVES	6*20	
WOOD CHOPS (UPPER PULLEY)	6*20	

DAY FOUR: ARMS / ABS	SETS * REPS	WEIGHT / EXERCISE
CLOSE GRIP PRESS	6*6,5,4,3,2,1	
CHIN UPS	6*6,5,4,3,2,1	
TRICEPS EXT.	6*6,5,4,4,4,4	
HAMMER CURLS (CABLE)	6*6,5,4,4,4,4	
PLANK (WEIGHTED)	5*60sec	

DAY FIVE: LEGS / ABS	SETS * REPS	WEIGHT / EXERCISE
FRONT SQUATS	6*6,5,4,3,2,1	
SUMO DEADLIFT	6*6,5,4,3,2,1	
FRONT RAISES	6*6,5,4,3,2,1	
RDL'S	6*6,5,4,3,2,1	
SEATED CALVES	6*20	
CABLE CRUNCHES	6*15	

HYPERTROPHY - WEEK 10 & 11 & 12

VOLUME 75% 1RM

REST 90sec - 150sec

FREQUENCY: 6x/Week

10 MINUTES DYNAMIC STRETCHES BEFORE TRAINING

AND 10 MINUTES STATIC AFTER TRAINING.

DAY ONE: PUSH	SETS * REPS	WEIGHT / EXERCISE
CHEST PRESS (BB)	6*8,8,8,6,6,4	
PUSH UPS	6*8 (3-1-3-1)	
FLYS (CABLE-MID PULLEY)	6*8	
CHEST PRESS (DB)	6*8	
KICK BACKS	6*8	
FRENCH PRESS (CABLE)	6*8	
REAR DELTS (MACHINE)	6*8	
HANGING LEG RAISES (WEIGHTED)	4*15	

DAY TWO: PULL	SETS * REPS	WEIGHT / EXERCISE
DEADLIFT	6*8,8,8,6,6,4	
LAT PULLDOWNS (WIDE GRIP)	6*8	
PULLOVER	6*8	
CONCENTRATED CURLS (CABLE)	6*8	
HAMMER CURLS	6*8	
SHRUGS (CABLE)	6*8	
FACE PULLS	6*8	
BACK EXTENSION	4*10	

DAY THREE: LEGS	SETS * REPS	WEIGHT / EXERCISE
BACK SQUATS	6*8,8,8,6,6,4	
GOBLET SQUAT w/ ISO HOLD (5sec)	6*8	
SPLIT SQUAT (NARROW) (smith)	6*8	
LEG PRESS	6*8	
SINGLE LEG EXT.	6*8	
UNILATERAL SEATED CALVES	6*10	
RUSSIAN TWISTS (WEIGHTED)	4*15	

DAY FOUR: PUSH	SETS * REPS	WEIGHT / EXERCISE
ARNOLD PRESSES	6*8,8,8,6,6,4	
LATERAL RAISE (CABLE)	6*8	
FRENCH PRESS (CHIN)	6*8	
FRONT RAISES	6*8	
OVERHEAD EXT (CABLE)	6*8	
DIPS	6*8	
CROSSOVER (LOW PULLEY)	6*8	
BICYCLE CRUNCHES	4*30	

DAY FIVE: PULL	SETS * REPS	WEIGHT / EXERCISE
ALT. BICEP CURLS	6*8	
E-Z BAR REVERSE CURLS	6*8	
CABLE CURLS	6*8	
GRIP ISOMETRIC	6*FAIL	
T-BAR ROWS	6*8,8,8,6,6,4	
ONE ARM ROWS	6*8	
BENT UNDER ROWS	6*8	
REVERSE CRUNCHES	4*12	

DAY SIX: LEGS	SETS * REPS	WEIGHT / EXERCISE
HIP THRUSTS	6*8,8,8,6,6,4	
RDL'S	6*8	
PULL THROUGHS	6*8	
GOOD MORNING	6*8	
LEG CURLS	6*8	
BOSU SQUATS	6*10	
UNILATERAL SEATED CALVES	6*8	
PLANK	4*60sec	

CONGRATULATIONS!

YOU DID IT!

You've just finished HERCULES WORKOUTS. Now you are ready to challenge yourself more and acquire more than you have previously thought possible!

You have come to a good muscular level and now it's time to think if you want to do another round of bulk training or if you want to do a round to get a cut on the weight you gained.

This will be done in another twelve weeks to acquire the body of Hercules and to accomplish all your daily labours.

We give you another two weeks of deload that you can follow if you want to have a relaxed training for 2 weeks, so you can recover better and avoid injuries from the training you just did.

The decision is yours. Whatever it is, share your experience with us and leave a comment on our page on Instagram for us to find out what you think of our program for bulk and muscular hypertrophy.

EXTRA

Therefore, for all of you who want something more and don't want these trainings to end, we have 2 extra weeks with less intensity and less Volume (sets-reps) so you can rest more properly. Training two or three times a week is just fine.

The ideal would be one training every 3 days. Because after all these trainings and all the stress that our muscles went through, we have to give them a little time to rest and get better.

You will see that as soon as you let your body go 4-5 days without training, it will seem firmer.

Your body will reward you in some way for letting it rest.

And after that, you will do 2 weeks of strength training from those we already have in our program and then the Upper - Lower protocol once again for 4 to 6 weeks.

Always stay concentrated, strong and tuned in on our page on Instagram that you will find at the end of this book.

DELOAD WEEK

VOLUME 55% 1RM

REST 120sec - 180sec

FREQUENCY: 3x/Week

10 MINUTES DYNAMIC STRETCHES BEFORE TRAINING

AND 10 MINUTES STATIC AFTER TRAINING.

DAY ONE: LEGS / DELTS	SETS * REPS	WEIGHT / EXERCISE
FRONT SQUATS	3*12	
LEG PRESS	3*12	
GLUTE BRIDGE	3*12	
FACE PULLS	3*12	
RUSSIAN TWISTS	3*12	
STANDING CALVES	3*12	

DAY TWO: BACK / TRICEPS / ABS	SETS * REPS	WEIGHT / EXERCISE
PULL DOWNS	3*12	
ONE ARM ROWS	3*12	
BENT OVER ROWS	3*12	
KICKBACKS	3*12	
BACK EXT.	3*12	
SEATED CALVES	3*12	

DAY THREE: CHEST / BICEPS / ABS	SETS * REPS	WEIGHT / EXERCISE
OVERHEAD PRESS (DB)	3*12	
FLYS (DB)	3*12	
PUSH UPS	2*12	
BICEP CURLS (DB)	3*12	
HAMMER CURLS	3*12	
PLANK	3*30sec	
STANDING CALVES	3*12	

About The Author

ACHILLEAS KARAKATSANIS is a certified personal trainer who loves fitness and a healthy nutrition lifestyle.

He lives in Athens and Santorini, Greece. Achilleas loves writing and reading books, watching and creating videos and inspiring his trainees to build their physique and a strong Mindset.

Make sure to watch our training videos in our page on

Instagram:

https://www.instagram.com/aka_achilles/

and feel free to contact us on:

achilleas.ebooks@hotmail.com

www.ingramcontent.com/pod-product-compliance
Lightning Source LLC
Chambersburg PA
CBHW031151250726
48655CB00002B/927